THE TSUNAMI DIET

Dr. Nathan H. Johnson

DISCLAIMER

The information and diet plan provided in this book is on an "as is" and "as available" basis. There is no representations or warranties of any kind, expressed or implied. Before starting any exercise or diet plan, a licensed physician or health care provider should be consulted. Failure to do so may result in harm or death. The concepts, ideas, ideas, and opinions expressed in this book are those of the author and no one else. This book, and information contained therein, is offered with the understanding that author is not rendering medical advice of any kind intended to replace medical advice, nor to diagnose, prescribe or treat any disease, condition, illness or injury. Again, it is imperative that before beginning any diet or exercise program, including any aspect of this book, you receive full medical clearance from a licensed physician. The Food and Drug Administration has not evaluated the statements contained in this book. If your healthcare provider has not cleared you to follow the exercise or nutritional concepts contained in this book, or if you have any hesitation whatsoever, disregard all information in this book.

ABOUT THE AUTHOR

Dr. Nathan Johnson has a Doctorate in toxicology and holds an advance certification in clinical chemistry. He has taken graduate level coursework in biochemistry, animal and human nutrition. Dr. Johnson's research interests include the effect of exercise and proper nutrition on healthcare utilization and longevity.

ACKNOWLEDGEMENTS

I would like to thank my family, friends, and co-workers for listening to my theories over the past 25 years. I would also like to thank my deceased father, a veterinarian, for discussing animal nutrition with me.

CHAPTER 1: INTRODUCTION

How many diet books have been written? A quick search on Amazon.com turns up over 100,000 titles. In other words, there is a unique diet book for every 2,000 or so adults in the United States. Does it have to be this complicated? I do not believe so. Please read this book with an open mind and understand that simple is good. This "diet" is not intended for rapid weight loss. It is intended for sustained weight loss. This "diet" is not intended to be hard to follow, rather, it is intended to be easily incorporated into daily life. I call this plan "The Tsunami Diet". Like a tsunami, this plan is powerful and your weight and body mass index will come crashing down over time. Once a tsunami is in motion, it is impossible to stop and you will see it coming! I truly believe this book may open the door to your "weight loss tsunami"! It should be noted that while this effort is based on science, I purposefully chose not to make this a "scientific work". For studies mentioned in this book, I will be happy to provide the appropriate references. In addition, I welcome your feedback and success stories. Please email me at tsunamidiet@gmail.com.

CHAPTER 2: WHY DIETS FAIL

Do you ever wonder why diets fail? Many people will blame the diet, but the real answer is in the mirror. Diets fail because humans implement the diet. We stop dieting because we are limited in the food we are allowed to eat, we get hungry, or the results do not seem like they are worth it. What if there was a diet plan where you never had to give up the foods you like to eat? What if there were no long periods of time where you "felt hungry"? What if you could stay on this diet no matter the social setting?

The tsunami diet will allow you to overcome all of the hurdles that always get in the way of dieting. Will it take effort on your part? Yes, but not the kind of effort that will feel overbearing. Are their rules to follow? Yes, but very simple rules that are easy to follow. Will you lose weight quickly? It depends on how "quick" is defined, but initial weight loss of one percent of body weight per week should be expected. Are you on-board? The next few chapters will describe the diet in detail.

CHAPTER 3: A PRIMER FOR SUCCESS

This book will not delve deeply into the biochemistry of nutrition. However, there are a few things that I think all individuals who are interested in weight loss need to know. Many readers will know most of what I will discuss and these points are very simple. However, as was previously mentioned, the intent of this diet is to keep it simple!

FACT #1: You need to eat to live. If you do not eat, you will die. If you must eat, then we should eat smartly.

FACT #2: Each of us has a different metabolism and lifestyle. No two individuals will get the exact same result from any change in diet and exercise. However, from epidemiology studies, we know that most individuals will respond in a similar manner. Our results will be distributed in a manner that will allow us to make predictions for the vast majority.

FACT #3: No two individuals have the same affinity for food. Our chance for success in any diet is increased if we like what we eat. This diet will allow you great choice in what you eat.

FACT #4: Most people do not understand how to read a nutritional label. Learning to read a nutritional label will help you in your weight loss journey.

FACT # 5: There are many low calorie alternatives to traditional high calorie choices.

FACT # 6: Smaller portions of high satiety foods, those that make you feel full, may be smarter than larger portions of lower calorie foods.

FACT #7: Short periods of fasting can be beneficial to your weight loss.

FACT #8: Those who measure their success/progress do better than those who don't.

CHAPTER 4: THE ONE WEIGHT LOSS PRINICPLE THAT NEVER FAILS

It took me many years to accept this simple fact of diet and nutrition. There are no shortcuts. Our bodies are designed in such a manner that increases our chances of survival. Did you ever wonder why some high calorie foods taste so good? Historically, those with some "reserve" tended to survive the hard times. Over the eons, these genes have been passed down to many of us. This genetic predisposition, along with the ease of good tasting, high calorie food, has created a double negative when it comes to keeping our weight in check. Top that with increasingly non-physical work, and it is easy to see why so many of us are overweight (body mass index >25%) or obese (body mass index >30%).

No matter what challenges we may have, in all but the most unusual of circumstances, you will lose weight if you expend more energy that you take in. There are some very basic terms and principles that you need to understand for all of this to make sense. You are probably familiar with the term "Calorie". In the scientific community, if you mention "Calorie", you are actually talking about 1/1000th of what we generally mean when discussing calories (kilocalorie). A kilocalorie is energy required to raise the temperature of a liter of water one degree centigrade at sea level. In the rest of the book, I will use the term calorie to actually mean kilocalorie. The main point is that a "calorie" represents an amount of energy.

When it comes to thinking about how our body uses energy, it is a good idea to think of our body like a furnace. Think of the amount of energy it would take to keep your house at a certain temperature if the conditions inside and the conditions outside never changed. There may be a little variation, but in general, it would take the same daily energy to keep the house at a constant temperature. Our bodies are the same way. If we did the exact same thing every day and our environment stayed the same, we would use the same amount of energy. Now, some of us have "big houses" and some have "little houses". Some have efficient furnaces and some have inefficient furnaces. This analogy is somewhat simplistic, but just understand that we each use a certain amount of energy just by being alive and doing nothing. The amount of energy we expend just by living is called our basal metabolic rate (BMR). There are many online calculators and below is just an example of one on the internet.

http://www.bmi-calculator.net/bmr-calculator/

Using this calculator, and inputting my age (47), height (76 inches) and current weight (220 pounds), I find that my BMR is 2082 calories. That means that if I do nothing else in life, and intake 2082 calories a day, in theory, I should maintain my current weight. There are many out there that make a living out of convincing people that the "kind of intake" is the secret. Depending on the person, there may some truth to that, but my strong belief is that we need to concentrate on the "intake" and "energy expenditure" no matter the source of each. If we do this right, we will lose weight.

The strongest argument supporting the simple math of weight loss comes from two types of data. The first comes from the hardships faced by humans over the years. The second comes from controlled animal trials. There are far too many of each to adequately address in this book, but I will highlight several.

The most direct observational evidence comes from data collected during times of famine and conflict. During conflicts such as the American Revolution and the Civil War, there have been no accounts of weight gain due to scarceness of food. In addition, in World War II, those held against their will and whose caloric intake did not meet their energy needs, all lost weight. The same principle has been shown when extreme environmental conditions exist. For example, when

Napoleon's Army invaded Russia during the mini-ice age, many starved to death in a combination of inadequate food intake and increased energy expenditure. You may also recall hearing about the extremely high caloric intake required by early humans and Neanderthals. I suspect that there were not many of these individuals chasing mammoths with a "beer belly".

Controlled animal studies also support universal weight loss by controlling caloric intake. The most cited studies go back to the 1930s and have been touted by the "caloric restriction" community. By the 1920s, science had advanced to using fairly robust animal models. In one particular experiment, the amount of food allocated to each rodent was drastically cut due to shortage of food and not by the design of the experiment. To the amazement of the researchers, the rodents lived longer than the normal two or so expected years. What was not a surprise to the researchers was that each of the animals lost weight! Current research conducted on non-human primates by the National Institute on Aging, part of the National Institutes of Health, and other similar studies by academic organizations continue to show that a dramatic reduction in caloric intake is indeed followed by weight loss.

I hope by this point you understand and agree that using more energy than what is consumed in calories is key to weight loss. If it is truly so easy, then why do we struggle with weight loss? In my opinion, we, as a society, need to make smarter choices. It is so easy to say eat less and exercise more! In reality, if we did just this, we would benefit greatly. What would happen if our overall caloric intake was reduced by just five percent and our energy expenditure was increased by just five percent? The results would be shocking....in a good way!

A good question to ask at this point....how do I eat less? Before we get to that question, let's go over just a few basics. Food intake is usually broken down into grams ingested. There are about 28 grams in an ounce and about 454 grams in a pound. Think about that the next time your order a one pound steak! There are three types of food that make up our caloric intake. They are carbohydrates, proteins, and fat. After rounding up and down, we consider each gram of carbohydrate and protein to yield four calories and each gram of fat to yield nine calories. This is why, pound for pound, the early humans got more bang for their buck when their meals included lots of fat!

It is very important to understand what proportion of the three types of food you are eating. If you eat a meal with lots of fat, you are actually eating "less" weight wise. Eating foods with more carbohydrates or protein will allow for more food per unit of weight. Fatty foods, while perhaps not always good for you, do provide some satiation or "feeling full". Proteins tend to provide more satiation than carbohydrates. Have you even eaten a high carb meal and shortly after feel hungry again? If so, you have just experienced a low satiation meal. Fiber has also been shown to provide some satiation. Everyone is different, so you may need to experiment.

The key, therefore, is to eat less than we you take in. Knowing what your BMR is, what you daily intake is, and how many additional calories you are burning is key. Attachment 1 is a simple worksheet to help you calculate how much weight you can lose given that you eat/exercise and expect to lose.

CHAPTER 5: THE MIRACLE OF OATMEAL

I have been a fan of oatmeal for as long as I can remember. It was a staple in my home when I was growing up. In the late 80s, I ate oatmeal as the American Heart Association touted its contributions to a "heart healthy diet" and possible contributions to lowering total cholesterol. I was an undergraduate student at the time and once ate oatmeal every morning for about six weeks. I must say I was disappointed at my results as I saw little change in my cholesterol. It was not until later in life that I realized the lack of dramatic change had more to do with the large number of other variables that affect cholesterol (see National Cholesterol Education Panel) than my eating oatmeal every day!

Despite my lack of "success", research has continued on the contributions of cholesterol to a healthy diet. This was vividly confirmed to me when a relative of mine made a dramatic change in their diet. This dietary change was made with very little change in exercise habits. The two biggest changes were the addition of fruits and vegetables (see Chapter 8) and daily consumption of a very large bowl of oatmeal. The average observer would dismiss adding a very large bowl of oatmeal to a weight loss plan. I would beg to differ. There are several advantages, both to health and weight loss, to a daily serving of oatmeal.

The first advantage to eating oatmeal daily is the mere fact of meal substitution. When you substitute a healthy option for a meal, which in effect means that one third of your meals are accounted for in a healthy fashion. In other words, you have one third less "opportunity" to have an unhealthy meal.

The second advantage to eating oatmeal daily is the satiation, or feeling of fullness that oatmeal gives you. There are many healthy additions to oatmeal such as berries and nuts that can add to this satiating feeling.

The third advantage to eating oatmeal daily is the long term health benefits. In addition to losing weight on the Tsunami Diet, you may also obtain health benefits. Oatmeal is a good source of Beta-glucans, a soluble fiber that has been shown to help lower total cholesterol. Oatmeal has also been shown to help keep glucose levels stable for extended periods which has many health benefits. Oatmeal is a good source of antioxidants and has also been shown to be a good way to naturally reduce your blood pressure. The high fiber content of oatmeal may decrease constipation and may aid in having a lower lifetime risk for colon cancer. Consistent consumption of oatmeal is often associated with a lower body weight, which can lead to many good health outcomes.

The final benefit of oatmeal is that it also makes a convenient between-meal snack. You can purchase individualized packages or you can make your own individual servings using bulk purchases of oatmeal and seal them in individual baggies. I have also frozen oatmeal in individual baggies with fresh fruit for a ready snack at a later date!

CHAPTER 6: CALORIE SUBSTITUTION

It is not hard to understand that the less you eat, the more weight you can lose. The problem is that the things many of us like to eat food that is very high in calories. Calorie substitution, that is substituting a high calorie food with a low calorie food, was the foundation for many of the early diets of the 1950s, 60s, and 70s. These diets, while showing initial promise, were long term failures with most who tried them. Why was this? There are a couple of reasons for this. First, the lower calorie food often tasted horrible. Second, this concept led to a daily calorie counting mentality that most people hate. Lastly, the variety of foods where there were calorie substitutes were minimal.

Today, there are many quality alternatives to high calorie foods. In fact, there are quite a few zero calorie substitutes. In the following portion of this Chapter, I will share with you some high caloric food substitutes. I have only chosen to include those that I have a first-hand knowledge of. In addition, I do not include substitutes that I believe are too expensive or not readily available.

Substitute # 1: Substitute low calorie (35 to 50 calories per slice) for high calorie bread (80 to 100 calories per slice). Also look at the fiber content. The higher the fiber, the better. Low calorie bread can be a great staple of the diet. You can eat it alone, make toast or French toast and make sandwiches.

Substitute # 2: Substitute lower calorie butter substitute for butter or margarine. There are many of these types of products on the market. My personal favorite and one that tastes the most like butter, at a very minimal calorie count, is "I Can't Believe It's Not Butter" spray.

Substitute # 3: Substitute deserts and snacks with vegetables and fruits. In addition to being healthy and adding fiber and critical anti-oxidants, vegetables and fruits will also limit the number of calories you consume.

Substitute # 4:   Substitute regular milk with low calorie soy milk. My favorite brand is soy slender and their chocolate milk has less than half the calories of whole milk.

Substitute # 5:   One of my very favorite low calorie food sources is actually a no calorie option! How can you top that? Walden farms makes a wide variety of zero calorie food substitutes. How? You will need to ask the folks at Walden farms that question, but their products are first rate. I have found the best prices at www.iherb.com Listed below are some of the food items that can be substituted with Walden farm products.

> *** Syrups – many flavors – my favorite!
> *** Cranberry Sauce
> *** Salad dressings
> *** BBQ Sauces
> *** Mayonnaise substitute
> *** Seafood sauce
> *** Ketchup
> *** Peanut Butter replacement (spread)
> *** Pasta Sauce
> *** Fruit spreads (jelly replacement)
> *** Fruit dips
> *** Chip dips
> *** Chocolate sauce
> *** Caramel Sauce

Substitute # 6:   No matter what type of food you like, there will be times when you honestly do not have time to prepare foods. It is for times like these that I like to always have a few lower calorie "TV dinners" available. The primary advantage of these meal options are portion control. You need to eat less and the manufacturer has an incentive to sell you less food for the same price, so it is a true "win-win". You need to watch what you buy as many of these dinners are very high in sodium and/or fat.

Substitute # 7:   If you routinely add sugar to your drinks or food, consider a low or no calorie sweetener substitute. The three major brands are Equal, Splenda, and Sweet and Low. Each of these brands has generic substitutions available.

Substitute # 8: If you are a drinker of soda, switching to a diet soda or low/no calorie water will save you a ton of calories of the course of a year. One of my favorite diet sodas is also very cheap, about 20 cents a can (diet GT Cola from Aldi).

Substitute # 9: In general, you can get many cuts of meat at a lower calorie count that normal. For instance, turkey bacon is but a fraction of what thick cut bacon might be. Another example, there are lower calorie bolognas (e.g. chicken bologna). In addition, there are vegetarian burgers, turkey sausage and other number of great tasting meat alternatives.

Substitute # 10: There are many varieties of low calorie popcorn. Skip the salt but load up on zero calorie spray butter. What something a little exotic? Try some popcorn coated with Walden Farms chocolate sauce that has been in the freezer for 30 minutes!

Substitute # 11: Although eggs are not that high in caloric content, you can save calories by using egg whites or egg substitute.

Substitute # 12: Salsa is a great low calorie alternative that goes great on many foods.

Substitute # 13: If you love soup, take a look at the caloric content. Many soups are actually very high in calories. Switch to canned broth based soups to reduce your caloric intake.

Substitute # 14: Ditch the French fries. Bake thinly sliced potatoes that have been sprayed with non-fat cooking spray. A little parmesan cheese on top and you have a great lower calorie alternative.

Substitute # 15: Do you like pasta but not the calories. Try shirataki noodles instead. These noodles are very low calories made from a type of yam. It is an acquired taste but many swear by it.

CHAPTER 7: ALTERNATE DAY CALORIC INTAKE

The real key to this diet is alternate day (ADD) caloric intake. Based on science that is almost 100 years old, alternate day dieting is a branch of the caloric restriction (CR) movement. CR has been shown to have a dramatic impact extending life expectancy and producing improvements in overall heath in many non-human life forms. While there is debate on the impact of CR on humans, there is no denying that adherence to a CR lifestyle produces weight loss. If you would like to see this for yourself, you can visit caloric restriction.org and you will see the results. The main obstacle with CR is maintaining the lifestyle. The vast majority of individuals can't maintain the CR lifestyle for one week, let alone a lifetime! For me, I would need to eat about 1,000 calories a day. That's just not going to happen.

In the past few years, there has been quite a bit of research into ADD. The basic research question was "if CR works so well, what would happen if someone did it half of the time"? The underlying premise also assumed that while individuals have great difficulty dieting for long periods, most could actually adhere to dieting one day at a time. In other words, tomorrow would always be a "non-diet" day. Studies have shown that ADD can reduce inflammation, improve cardiovascular health, and results in weight loss. My own personal experience is that ADD works and the body of scientific work supports this.

I will not go into detail about ADD in this book, you can get that from other sources. In practice, you will actually eat a little more on days you are not dieting and should aim to much less on days you are dieting. For me, I aim for about 1,000 calories a day when I on my diet day and a little more than that if I am actively exercising. I do not even count calories on the day I am not dieting. Attachment 2 shows a calculation of the number of calories an individual might "save" in a year by following ADD.

CHAPTER 8: ADD A SPLASH OF VEGETARIAN

In the practice of alternate day dieting, there are some strategic things you can do to potentially accelerate the weight loss and health benefit process. One quick way to do this involves a bit of psychology. Although you should not count calories on the day you are not dieting, it would be great if you also ate a little less on those days. However, if you did that purposefully, you would essentially be moving toward a CR lifestyle, one that is not sustainable and leads to discouragement. We need a better way and one that "tricks" your mind!

A vegetarian diet is one that also yields many beneficial effects. It is also one that is hard for most to adhere to, although it is not as hard a CR. Personally, I love to eat meat, yet I often realize that I have went thru a whole day without eating any meat. For example, I may have oatmeal for breakfast, pasta for lunch, an apple for a mid-day snack, and a baked potato for dinner with vegetables. Without knowing it, I was a vegetarian for that day. Using this type of example, it seems that eating like this on your non-diet day makes a lot of sense. In addition to the benefits of ADD, you would also get some of the same benefits of eating a vegetarian diet, such as improved blood cholesterol levels, a healthy BMI, and lower rates of heart disease, stroke, diabetes, cancer, proved blood pressure, and longer life span. Since by nature these types of food are lower in calories, you can actually eat a greater volume that results in fewer calories. It is interesting that some of the same benefits of CR and ADD are the same benefits of a vegetarian diet. Therefore, if you ate vegetarian on your non-diet days, you are in effect supercharging your weight loss and getting additional health benefits.

CHAPTER 9: FIBER, ANTI-OXIDANTS, AND OTHER FUN STUFF

There are a few other items that you need to keep in mind while on this diet. First, you need to make sure that you eat an adequate amount of fiber per day. This can be an issue on the days you are dieting, especially if you eat a significant amount of meat on your diet day. Your daily oatmeal will provide you with a good start in getting enough fiber. Females need about 30 grams of fiber per day and males about 40 grams. How do you get to this level? My thought is that natural is always better, but if not, there are fiber supplements you can get, some of which are sugar free.

Anti-oxidants are also something you need to get from any diet. Since this diet should result in reduced caloric intake, we need to make sure we are not reducing anti-oxidants. What are anti-oxidants? They are any substance that inhibit the oxidation of other molecules. Chemically, in our body, oxidation can generate "free radicals" which can cause damage or death of a cell. Anti-oxidants inhibit oxidation by being oxidized themselves. You can think of anti-oxidants as the reserve force our body needs when oxidation gets out of control. There is still a much debate on the actually physiological benefit of anti-oxidant intake, but the reality is that these foods also have other benefits, so it is a good idea to target anti-oxidant rich foods in your diet. You can get some benefit from taking vitamins, but the best antioxidants come from healthy foods. There are many lists on the internet that categorize anti-oxidant rich food. In general, fruits, berries, nuts, and some vegetables are rich in anti-oxidants. Meat is low in anti-oxidants.

If you are inclined to eat a high fat diet on your "diet day", then you may also consider the use of the over the counter lipase inhibitor "Alli". Lipase is a naturally occurring enzyme that our body uses to break down fats in our intestine. Alli works to bind lipase. The end result is some fats are not broken down into absorbable free fatty acids. The selective use of Alli can result in a small decrease in the number of calories absorbed and it helps if your fiber intake is not adequate as it serves as a mild laxative and stool softener. There are definitely some negative side effects of Alli which include non-absorption of fat soluble vitamins (Vitamins A, D, E and K) and anal leakage of fat.

CHAPTER 10: EXERCISE – THE CHERRY ON TOP OF YOUR NEW LIFESTYLE

Exercise is not required for this diet to work. However, that does not mean that you should not exercise. There are many good reasons to exercise, here are a few which augment The Tsunami Diet very nicely.

First and foremost, exercise will increase the number of calories you can intake each day and remain at the same net caloric intake. That alone is a great reason to exercise. The second reason is that it clears your mind. The psychological benefits of exercise extend far beyond the exercise period. As a natural mood enhancer, consistent exercise will make staying on any diet plan easier. A third benefit of exercise is the well documented improvements to cardiovascular health and cholesterol levels. Are you noticing a trend here? You see the same benefit in many other chapters. Finally, exercise can lead to better, more consistent sleep! No more midnight snacks! One last thought, you can easily convert an old-treadmill into a "treadmill desk" where you can exercise while doing daily activities.

CHAPTER 11: EATING ON A BUDGET

The Tsunami Diet can actually be good for your bottom line as well. Think about it. You will be consuming fewer calories than before. That should equate to spending less on food. Oatmeal should be a staple of your daily diet. Oatmeal is dirt cheap. You will eat a vegetarian diet every other day. Generally, this is cheaper than a meat based diet. When eating out, meat is generally the most expensive component of the meal. The only more expensive part of this diet, if you choose to use them, are the low and zero calorie food replacements. You can choose to buy some of your items at low priced stores like Aldi as well or buy in bulk when particular items are on sale.

CHAPTER 12: NATE'S AMAZING "SUBSTITUTION" RECIPIES

The most amazing part of the Tsunami Diet is you can tailor it to eat the kind of foods you like. Below are a couple of the things I like to eat on this diet. You can really eat whatever you like. Is there a particular diet shake or product you like? You can easily plug and play into this diet. The sky is the limit. A sample of a two day diet is found at Attachment 3.

RECIPIE # 1: Apple Cinnamon Oatmeal

0.33 Cup Oatmeal
0.5 Cup Water
0.5 teaspoon ground cinnamon
Cubed apple – to taste
0.5 Cup Milk

Mix oatmeal, water, cinnamon and then microwave on high for 1 minute and 20 seconds. Add milk and apple and microwave for 10 seconds.

RECIPIE # 2: Low Calorie French Toast

4 Eggs or equivalent egg substitute
1 Dash cinnamon
4 slices of low calorie bread

Beat eggs in large bowl. Add dash of cinnamon. Coat bread with mixture. Cook on medium heat until brown on each side. Serve with Walden Farms zero calorie syrup of your choice. Sweeten with no calorie sweetener.

RECIPIE # 3: Low Calorie Frozen Treat

1 Frozen Peeled Banana
2 Tablespoons of Walden Farms Chocolate Syrup
2 Packages no calories sweetener
1.5 Cup of Soy Slender Chocolate Soy Milk
3 Tablespoon of Walden Farm Peanut Butter Spread
1.5 Cup of Ice Cubes

Blend all ingredients until smooth consistence

RECIPIE #4: Quick Banana Treat

1 Banana
4 Table Spoon Walden Farm Caramel Syrup
Regular whipped cream…not the creamy higher calorie version

Put banana in microwavable safe plate. Top with syrup and microwave for 40 seconds. Top with whip cream

RECIPIE #5: Low Cal PBJ Sandwich

2 Slices low calorie bread
Mixture of half peanut butter and Walden Farm Peanut Butter spread
Walden Farm zero calorie fruit spread, flavor of your choice

Spread mixture of peanut butter and spread with fruit spread onto bread. You can do this with either one or two slices. Enjoy!

RECIPIE #6: Low Cal Tuna Sandwich

2 Slices low calorie bread
Tuna Fish – amount is your choice
Walden Farm zero calories mayonnaise spread
Pickles, chopped
Onions (optional)

Combine all ingredients and spread onto bread

ATTCHMENT ONE: SIMPLE WIEGHT LOSS CALCULATOR

Current Height_____ Age_____ Weight_____

BMR _____kCal/day

Extra Exercise _____ kCal/day

Total Expenditure per day (add previous two lines) _____

Calories Breakfast _____ kCal

Calories Lunch _____ kCal

Calories Dinner_____ kCal

Calories Snacks_____ kCal

Total Calories_____ kCal

Total Calories/day subtracted from Total Expenditure _____

If this number is positive, you have a negative balance (e.g. using more than you intake....this is good!!!)

ATTCHMENT TWO: SAMPLE CALORIC INTAKE USING ALTERNATE DAY DIET

	kCal Intake
Diet Day	1200
Non Diet Day	2500
Normal Day	2300
kCal for diet/per week	12950
kCal for normal/week	16100
	kCal
Difference Per Week	3150
Difference per Month	13650
Difference per Year	163800

ATTCHMENT THREE: SAMPLE TWO DAY DIET

DAY 1: ~1200 calories
Breakfast – Coffee with skim milk, oatmeal
Snack – Low calorie (100 calorie snack)
Lunch – Low calorie PBJ one or two
Snack – Apple
Dinner – Chicken Breast with Broccoli

DAY 2: ~2500 calories
Breakfast – Coffee with skim milk, oatmeal
Snack – Low calorie (100 calorie snack)
Lunch – Hamburger, Fries
Snack – Orange
Dinner – 6 oz steak, baked potato, small salad

NOTES PAGE

NOTES PAGE

NOTES PAGE